HOW TO GET ALONG WITH YOUR CO-WORKERS

LEARN HOW TO DEAL WITH THE PEOPLE YOU WORK WITH, ACTIVITIES TO IMPROVE WORKING

Gaston Echevarria

Table of Contents

Introduction

Probably more people than you think spend most of their time working with others in an employment-related situation. And, unless they're lucky, these individuals can't choose who their coworkers are.

Unfortunately, not everyone knows how to get along with others. This can cause all kinds of difficult situations, making it almost impossible to get through the day.

Working well with others is crucial in any situation. However, it is even more important in a working environment. Why is that? It comes down to things like efficiency, productivity and employee morale... just to name a few.

The size of the company or business you really work for doesn't matter. The rules are basically the same whether you work with someone else or 1,000 people. Each individual deserves the same level of consideration.

During your job search, have you ever noticed the phrase "should work well with others" in the job description or application? If so, there's a very good reason for it. Employers do not want to hire individuals who do not work well with others. Typically causes problems from the beginning.

Definition of others

In this case, "others" can be defined as all the people you come into contact with during work. Obviously, the answer is going to be different for everyone. However, it can include the boss, your co-workers, the customers or clients you interact with, any supplier you use, the HR team, maintenance or cleaning.... staff - the list goes on.

One of the main reasons why it is so important to treat everyone equally is that you never know what a person might help you or do for you in the future. Of course, that means never taking advantage of that particular person's assistance or eagerness to help, under any circumstances.

Are you familiar with the expression "it's not what you know, it's who you know"? Think of it this way. Someone you don't interact with on a daily basis, but still consider a friendly acquaintance, might share some advice with you regarding a friend you're hiring for a position you'd love to have. Without that advice, you wouldn't realize the opportunity. This scenario happens much more than you probably think. Just another reason to be considerate of everyone.

Another possibility is to make a friend you wouldn't otherwise have. Diversity in the workplace is more common than ever. This gives individuals a much better opportunity to make friends with someone who is not part of their daily life. It could be someone who works in a different department or the person who maintains the office grounds. When it comes to meeting and making a new friend, the possibilities are almost endless.

Why it can be difficult to work with others

There are several reasons why it can be difficult to work with others. Many people have a tendency to bring their egos to their workplace. It may be that these individuals are really self-conscious and unsure of themselves within. So, they use a big ego as a cover.

Honestly, the grandiloquence in the work turns against most of the time. It creates resentment and bad feelings very quickly. When an employee does not work well with others, for whatever reason, the chances of that person ending up being fired are high.

If this inappropriate behavior continues, the same person runs the risk of being fired over and over again until they finally find a job in which it doesn't matter to get along with people. It's a sad scenario when you think about it. Don't let it happen to you!

Another challenging part of working with others is making an effort to avoid competition. If a co-worker doesn't get along with you, it may be because of the competitive aspects of your job description and the fact that they are trying to beat you at something.

Yes, it is true that a little friendly competition can attract workers to improve their performance. However, raising another person's job performance to get to her is going to do nothing more than hurt her feelings. This can lead to a decline in your own performance and may even make you think about going ahead and finding a job elsewhere.

The importance of respect

If everyone at work isn't being treated with respect, it can be bad for business. If you do not feel that you are being treated with respect at work, it can be extremely difficult to do the best you can. The same goes for your co-workers. They may not be able to perform their duties efficiently if and when a disrespectful co-worker has compromised their confidence.

Mutual respect between workers also helps to foster an atmosphere of cooperation among team members. If you respect the people you work with, it is much easier to work with them to achieve a goal. If you don't have any respect for your co-workers or their skills, why would you count on them to help you?

The best way for a team of employees to build a bond of mutual respect is through training and exercises designed to help everyone get to know their co-workers and their skills. It can be as simple as having each team member share their name and the parts of their work where they feel best.

In an environment where disrespectful behavior is common, conflict between you and your co-workers is more likely to break out. But it's important not to let disrespectful behavior affect you and make you act the same way.

A conflict at work has a negative impact on both morale and overall productivity. If you feel that a co-worker is not treating you with respect, talk to him or her about your behavior in a calm and respectful manner. If you are not willing to discuss it, take the matter to your boss or supervisor.

Essential skills and habits you need to work with others

There are many essential skills and habits that you need to work well with others. Developing the right habits, from the beginning, helps steer you toward things like a higher salary and leadership opportunities. As more and more companies are making the decision to hire within the company, these things are more important than ever.

Many of these things will probably seem obvious to you. However, if they were obvious to everyone, they would not need to be listed. Keep in mind that this isn't a complete list of the skills and habits you need to succeed, but it definitely gives you a good starting point. As you can probably see, many of these suggestions don't require much more effort than remembering them. There's no reason to panic and think you have to change your whole lifestyle.

While these things may seem insignificant when looked at separately, not doing several of them adds up to a larger problem. It can really mean the difference between keeping a job and getting fired. This is especially true in today's economy. With so many people actively seeking employment, employers generally find it very easy to fill their vacancies.

Taking responsibility

It's always important to take responsibility for the things you do, especially when something goes wrong. Nobody's perfect. All but a few unrealistic employers realize that. If you make a mistake and claim it wasn't your fault, not only are you not telling the truth, but you're also giving the impression that you weren't in control of the situation.

When you take responsibility, you'll probably notice two things. First, your co-workers are likely to be more willing to help you correct the problem and help you succeed. Second, these same individuals will feel more comfortable around you, knowing that you are honest and that you will never blame anyone else.

> ***Keep an open mind***

Even in situations where you know you are 100 percent right, it is always advisable to keep an open mind. This is especially true when you are in a managerial position. Why is that? If you are never open to new ideas or alternatives, you may encounter someone who knows everything. When this happens, people get defensive very quickly and from there it's downhill.

It is much more productive to show a little humility and concern for really finding the right answer to every problem and situation. Because each person has a different problem-solving process, teamwork really has the potential to solve problems and generate great ideas much faster.

➢ *Deliver on Your Commitments*

Always try to give enough time to complete projects in a timely manner, even when something unexpected comes up. It is much better to give yourself more time than you need to finish each time you are working, rather than underestimating the time needed to complete the task. That way, you don't have to worry about disappointing your employer or colleagues.

Make an extra effort. Always keep track of things, whenever possible. This accomplishes two things. First, it strengthens relationships in the workplace. Second, it gives you important information about your performance.

➢ *Practice proper hygiene*

Regardless of whether you are working with the public or in an office, practicing proper hygiene is essential when you work with others. No one wants to be around someone who smells bad or seems to have slept in their clothes. This doesn't mean you have to dress like the rich and famous. It simply means showering daily and coming to work with a presentable look and smell.

If you have a limited budget, consider buying clothes at local thrift stores. You can pick up great deals on clothes that are perfectly suited for the job. These stores usually stock a wide variety of business suits at fantastic prices. You just have to be there at the right time, which is on the days when the store receives deliveries.

> ### ➢ *Turn your phone off*

Almost everyone has a cell phone these days. If you work in a large office, constant ringing can be a great distraction. Unless you need your phone for work purposes, turn it off or put it away. Quickly reading a text message when someone is talking to you is extremely rude. It gives the impression that your phone is more important than your job. Get in the habit of checking your messages or making quick calls during breaks or lunch.

> ## ➢ *Share Credit*

When applicable, sharing credit with your co-workers is a sure sign that you work well with others. Not only that person or individuals like you even more than they did before, you will probably earn a higher level of respect as well.

On the other hand, if you don't share credit when it's due, you'll earn a reputation as someone who is selfish and wants to sabotage everyone else in an attempt to get ahead. If you get away with it without anyone complaining, don't waste time celebrating. In reality, the truth usually prevails and you are not going to get ahead - you may be in line for the unemployed.

> ***Don't interrupt***

Have you ever been in the middle of a conversation, just to be constantly interrupted? It's annoying, isn't it? For that reason, never be the one who interrupts. Even if you have a great idea that you can't wait to share, wait until it's your turn to talk. Take a deep breath and relax. You'll share your news or ideas before you know it.

Here's a little secret. There are individuals who are not so impressed when you talk, no matter how fantastic your idea is. These people prefer to talk about themselves. So, when you let them talk first, it's a good way to make them love you. After that, they may be more receptive to what you say.

> **Smile**

The act of smiling is often referred to as a person's most powerful gesture. Science can support the fact that individuals who smile are often not only happier, but also more successful. Better yet, smiling doesn't cost you a penny. It's free to smile and see how the world (or at least the people you work with) gives you back your smile.

It is interesting to note that some training modules for customer service positions related to the phone require agents to keep a small mirror next to their phone. This way, the agent can make sure they are smiling when they talk to the client. Believe it or not, the person on the other side of the receiver can usually hear the smile in the agent's voice. This makes the interaction between the two much more pleasant and sales many times greater.

➢ *Use resources*

Working well with others, to the best of your ability, sometimes involves the use of resources. Depending on where you work and your job description, many companies offer all kinds of options for you to take advantage of.

These resources can be things like seminars, training sessions, fitness programs, free safety equipment, mental health and family counseling, and more. If you come across a good resource that you think would benefit your work environment and your co-workers, don't hesitate to mention it to your manager or boss. Who knows? You may even get a small reward or bonus for taking the initiative to recommend something that could help your business succeed.

> ### ➤ *Don't make noise*

If your employer allows you to listen to music or something similar, don't make noise. Use headphones or keep the volume at a level that won't distract you. Remember, not everyone will have the same musical taste as you. If your co-workers don't like what they hear, it will probably be harder for them to concentrate and do their job correctly. The time to make noise is after the work day is over, unless you are a rock musician or an auctioneer.

➢ *Respect the limits*

Your job may require you to share a space with your co-workers, whether it's a cubicle, an office or a vehicle. If you are close to others while working, be sure to respect their limits and encourage them to respect yours in return.

Try not to get phone calls about non-work related issues if your cubicle partner is quietly focused on a project. Also, try not to disclose too much about your personal life, because this may be too much information for some people. These limits will differ from person to person, so if you're not sure if your behavior will bother your co-worker, it may be best to ask first.

> ### ➤ *Learn to let go*

Once you have had a dispute with a co-worker, it may be difficult for your relationship with him or her to return to a state where you can work together effectively. If the dispute has been resolved, the best thing you can do is focus on the job. Of course, your co-worker will have to concentrate on letting go as well.

If they still seem upset about it, see if they're willing to talk about it. If they tell you why they are still not satisfied after the dispute has been resolved, do what you can to fix things between the two of you. If problems persist between the two of you, it is best to inform your boss or supervisor.

Benefits of Working Effectively with Others

Teamwork is a wonderful thing. It may take everyone a little time to get into the vibe. But when that happens, it's beneficial to everyone involved, not to mention the company's success. These are some of the benefits of working together at work. Yes, it can be done!

✓ **Fills Voids**

Working together typically fills gaps. Not everyone has the same skills or education. Teamwork allows people to contribute their own knowledge to a project or problem as a whole.

It's also very useful when someone is sick. If no one jumps to do that person's job, everything could stop until the employee feels well enough to go back to work. Businesses lose business when they operate at less than 100 percent.

✓ **Promotes Healthy Competition**

There is absolutely nothing wrong with a little healthy competition in the workplace. This often leads to an increase in productivity, which is always encouraged. He's also an excellent motivator. Many times, when co-workers see their co-workers doing an excellent job, they want to do everything possible to match (or even exceed) performance.

✓ **Encourages conflict resolution**

No matter how well you and your teammates work together as a group, there is always the possibility of conflict from time to time. There is no guarantee that they can be avoided altogether. This is partly due to the fact that employees come from different backgrounds and have different styles of doing things. It's what makes the world and the work environment so interesting.

When conflicts arise, your team is forced to find the solution that best suits the situation. This is a very good skill to have on hand, especially for those interested in future promotional opportunities.

✓ **Inspires risk taking**

You may not think that taking risks is

something you should try at work. However, there is something like "healthy" risk-taking. Think of it this way. If you were working on a project on your own and that project failed in some way, you would be responsible for the failure in its entirety.

On the other hand, if you are working in a team, your co-workers not only share ideas, but also the success or failure of the final result. In essence, teamwork gives everyone in the group the freedom to think safely outside the box and really think of new possibilities.

✓ **Increases efficiency**

The more effectively a team of employees works, the more work they can do. Of course, having more people means being able to make more effort. But, one big team can actually stand in the other's way if they're not working together effectively. Even if you don't work directly with a team, effective communication with other members of your organization helps get things done as quickly as possible.

✓ **Establishes Trust**

Finishing a project with co-workers does a lot to build a relationship with them. Once they help you do things, you'll know that you can trust them again in the future. This sense of confidence will give you a level of security that will make it much easier to work and share ideas with your co-workers.

On the other hand, if team members don't trust each other, they can make decisions that aren't good for business in the long run. They may feel that they are the only members of the team who can do the work and therefore try to do it all themselves. This could lead to a serious drop in efficiency, and potentially even greater problems if the added stress causes this employee to make a mistake.

Training of new employees

If you are in charge of training new employees in the workplace, it will have a big impact on your impression of the organization as a whole. If your training is effective, and you are there to help them when they need you, they will see that the company is useful and a good place to work. But if you don't give them the help they need, they're unlikely to establish a positive relationship with the company. Here are a few things to keep in mind as you train a new employee.

> ➢ *Focus on building strengths*

As you work with a new employee, be aware of the areas in which they excel and encourage them to take advantage of their experience. This will not only encourage them to do a good job now, but will also prepare them to get a promotion for a job that suits their skills in the future. Also, ask them if they have other strengths that can help them get the job done. They can help the company in ways you hadn't thought of beforehand.

> ***Find online resources (as you are doing now)***

There are a number of different learning programs available on the Internet that are well suited to many different companies and organizations. These courses typically include written instructions and instructional videos, as well as interactive components such as quizzes, puzzles, or even games. With such a wide variety of courses available, you are required to find a course for each department in your organization. All it takes is a little research.

➢ *Ask for help*

If you have difficulty training new employees, it may be time to call for help. Workplace vocational training companies are out there and can help educate their staff on a large number of things.

Typically, these groups come directly to your workplace to administer your training. However, the assistance provided can be quite costly. To minimize training costs, think of your current staff. If any of them have exceptional talent in one of the areas covered by your training, ask them if they would be willing to spend any time with your students. They may be able to provide ideas that would not have occurred to you.

> ***Encourage learning***

It's hard to teach someone who doesn't want to hear what you have to say. And, if your new employees aren't enthusiastic about their new job, it can be difficult to train them to do things effectively.

It is important that you arouse interest in your apprentice so that he or she learns about your work, rather than simply telling you what to do. Make sure they know there's nothing wrong with asking questions, even if it's less about their work and more about the company as a whole. The more motivated they are to learn, the better their performance will improve over time.

Give them something to make it happen.

After you have instructed your new employee on how to do their job, give them something to do so they can see how much of their training they can remember. Be sure to watch them as they do, but try not to interfere too much unless they need help. Not only does it give you a good idea of what they have learned, but it will also help them find ways to apply it to their new job and help them have a sense of accomplishment.

✓ **Keep the fun**

One of the most important things you can do to help build a relationship between your apprentice and your organization is to keep the tone light and friendly. This does not mean that you should make your training less effective, or that you should not work as hard during the training period. Just be sure to smile and keep things positive while working with them. Not only will it make learning their new job more enjoyable for them, but socializing with them now could also lead to making a new friend in the future.

✓ **Types of workplace conflicts**

Like conflicts in our personal lives, workplace conflicts can be difficult to avoid. Disputes between co-workers are often resolved between the parties involved without problems. However, it may sometimes be necessary to contact your human resources department or senior management to resolve the problem if the conflict cannot be resolved.

Part of managing conflicts effectively is knowing what kind of workplace conflict you are dealing with when the problem arises.

✓ **Leadership**

A change in leadership, such as a new supervisor or managerial staff, can cause major conflicts among employees. A sudden change in leadership can take some getting used to and can be stressful for you and your co-workers in the process.

Drastic changes in leadership at work take people out of their comfort zone as they try to adjust to new rules and techniques, all while maintaining their workload. Although at first it may seem daunting, much of this conflict can be avoided by providing a clear summary of any changes being made to workplace rules.

✓ **Conflicts of character**

Personality conflicts are some of the most common problems among co-workers. It can be difficult to grasp the social cues you're not used to, or to understand the mannerisms that differ from yours and the people you're in regular contact with. It is best to try not to take things so personally to avoid unnecessary confrontations.

If you can't think of a reason why your colleague is acting negatively towards you, you may have noticed something that wasn't there. It is very unlikely that

your co-worker would arbitrarily decide to
be rude to you.

It is easier to change oneself than to change others

Typically, change for the better is not easy for anyone to achieve. You can't just snap your fingers or wave a magic wand and expect those changes to happen overnight. But think how great it would be if it were really possible to accomplish the task!

However, keep this in mind. Although it is possible to change oneself (with a little effort - sometimes more than one is willing to put into it), it is extremely difficult to change others. Moreover, when you take the time to think about it, do you really have that right?

It's hard to change a situation where

you don't have a record and all the facts. It's the same with a person. Until you've walked in someone's shoes, you don't know why that person acts the way they do. You may have a general idea, but generalities are not enough.

Whether you're at work or somewhere else, whenever you feel like changing someone, try this instead. Think of things YOU can do to improve the issue. Going out and telling someone that you think you need to change is a safe way to start bad feelings between the two of you. Honestly, how would you feel if things changed and someone told you that you needed to alter the way you do things?

A good example of this is time management. You notice that one of your co-workers is finding it difficult to meet the timeline regarding the completion of a project. Instead of going to your manager with a complaint, why not ask the boss if there's any way to help the individual stay on the right track? You may even learn something new in the process.

If someone wants to change and asks you for help, it's something completely different. Doing everything possible to help them will help ensure the transformation they hope to achieve. Sometimes, all individual needs are a push in the right direction. Look at it this way: they'd probably do the same for you.

> ***When to call the boss***

Many interpersonal conflicts at work can be resolved without management being involved. Your co-workers are adults, and you should be able to reach a reasonable outcome for any dispute you may have. While it's a good idea to keep your boss informed about what's going on between you and your co-workers, going to them with every issue can lead your co-workers to believe that you're not willing to listen to their side of the story.

However, if neither of you wants to compromise on the issue, it may be a good idea for a supervisor or HR representative to meditate on the conflict for you. Set a time when everyone can meet to solve the problem. With a neutral party involved to listen to both sides of the story, they may be more inclined to stop any behavior that is causing a problem.

➢ *Introverted Works*

If you are an introvert, you can still take advantage of the guidance offered in this report. You just won't have to depend on him so often. If you are the shy type, consider applying for the following type of work. If you don't find one right away, don't give up. They're out there.

> ***Animal care***

If you like animals, think about getting a job in a veterinarian's office, an animal shelter, or even a pet store. Although pay is lower than many other employment opportunities, most of the time is spent working with animals. Leave interaction with humans to your extroverted co-workers.

> ***Social Media Manager***

At first, this may seem like a strange choice. Yes, work requires interacting with people. But since everything is done over the Internet, you don't have to be face to face with the people you're communicating with. With the growing popularity of social platforms, it is likely that there is always a need for this behind-the-scenes management position.

➢ *Court Reporter*

At the time of writing, the Bureau of Labor Statistics indicates that the average income of a court reporter is only $50,000 per year. Although a court reporter is required to be in the courtroom, he or she has very little interaction with anyone. The only time that speech is required is when someone asks the individual to read part of the court transcript.

➢ *Freelance Writer*

Thanks to the popularity of the Internet, opportunities for freelance writing seem to be everywhere. Better yet, you don't need a college degree to get started. If you can write in an interesting way and have a basic knowledge of grammar, customers are out there waiting for your help.

Typically, the only time you have to interact with someone is when you are talking about a possible job or have questions for a current client. Even then, almost anything can be done via email.

> ***Translator***

If you speak one or more foreign languages, why not make additional use of these skills? The job of a translator is simply to convert written documents or audio recordings from one language to another. No additional participation of co-workers is required.

Other possible options, with limited human interaction, include the following:

- Truck driver or dealer
- Security Guard
- Counter
- Landscaper
- Concierge
- Laboratory technician or researcher
- Artist
- Graphic Designer

For more ideas, take an hour or so to do an online search. You'll probably be surprised by job suggestions for people who prefer to limit interaction with co-workers.

Conclusion

This information is just a small sampling of the things you can do to make sure you always work well with others, regardless of your job description or the position you hold in the company. Obviously, the easier it is for you to interact with your co-workers and customers, the greater the chances of getting a raise or promotion.

You may have to work on some of these things before they start to feel natural. The good news is, if that's the case, it's totally fine. Don't punish yourself for that. There is no such thing as a perfect employee, no matter how much education or experience in the field he or she has.

In any job, two of the most important

traits to possess are diligence and honesty. As long as you exhibit these two qualities, it is very likely that you will succeed and, better yet, that you will feel good about doing so.

Just as there is no perfect employee, there is no perfect job or set of co-workers. There will probably be times when you feel frustrated by both, which is perfectly natural. During those periods, do everything you can to stay positive about the situation.

Being positive is a decision you make. It doesn't just depend on the good things that happen to you. If you remain positive even when things aren't the best, your co-workers will be more likely to notice your attitude and try to match it.

Some people are more introverted and

prefer to work alone. If you fall into this category, that's fine too. As long as you can find a job you like to do, that's the most important thing. However, you may want to consider this. By practicing some of the suggestions in this report, you may gradually find yourself a little more extroverted.

If that happens and you feel more comfortable with people, it may be time to try to broaden your career horizons. This new sense of confidence won't happen overnight. But, with practice in patience, you may eventually find yourself wanting to work with others. And there's certainly nothing wrong with that.

Just remember that everything will not happen overnight and that it will take time before you see a change in your life for the better.

Now yes, I wish you the best in your results, and remember, everything is practical; theory without action is of no use to you. It brings everything you learn into real life.

A big hug, your friend, Gaston!

By the way, when you achieve your results little by little, I highly recommend you, if you want to improve your social skills, I highly recommend you, the book of a great friend of mine, on "HOW TO CONTROL SOCIAL ANSIETY AND PANIC ATTACKS", is a book that I'm sure will help you a lot to avoid any kind of anxiety. Without further ado, you can find it in the Amazon search engine, such as: "How to control social anxiety and panic attacks" or looking for its name, such as: "Jorge O. Chiesa"... Once again I wish you success in your results!

www.ingramcontent.com/pod-product-compliance
Lightning Source LLC
Chambersburg PA
CBHW071239240726
48654CB00009B/1128